Fifty S

MW01488940

Laina Charleston

Married Sex
Fifty Shades of Grey for Couples
© 2012 by Laina Charleston

This book is licensed for your personal enjoyment only.

WARNING: EXPLICIT SEXUAL CONTENT! ADULTS ONLY

You must be 18 years of age to read the contents.

PREFACE

Unleash your inner goddess...

Has reading Fifty Shades of Grey spiked your interest in the world of BDSM? You don't need a red room of pain when a nightstand drawer of pleasure will do. Go from mild to wild with a checklist of all things naughty from Fifty Shades. With helpful hints FOR HIM and FOR HER, the sexual behaviors from the trilogy are condensed into an easy to implement couple's guide for a more satisfying sex life. From the erotic touch of a lover's massage to the tingling feel of a good spanking, this book gets to the nitty gritty brought to light by the worldwide phenomenon. Everything you need to go from demure diva to sexy siren with over 115 ways to increase your threshold of pleasure. Select just two ideas a week and you've got an entire year of kinky sex to enhance the action between your sheets.

Married Sex: Fifty Shades of Grey for Couples

PART ONE: Sensual Intimacy

Sensual Massage
Rub a Dub in the Tub
Mirror, Mirror
Email Me
Shave Me
Silky Hair
Shower Sex
Making Out
Satin Sheets
Mutual Masturbation
Pin Me Down
Taste Me
Cover My Eyes
Kissing

PART TWO: Roughin' It

PART THREE: Kinky Fuckery

Sir or Mistress
Anal Plug
Anal Beads
Nipple Clamps
Genital Clamps
Wartenberg Pinwheel
Ball Gag
Spreader Bar
Riding Crops
Period Sex
Ben Wa Balls
Tie Me Up
Vibrators

SENSUAL INTIMACY

This first part of the book focuses on the more sensual aspects of lovemaking. Things you did when you were first dating, but over the years have been pushed aside. Ideas range from easygoing to slightly kinky where both partners will probably stay within their comfort zones. Ease into your kinky side with any one of the milder ideas presented in Fifty Shades; adapted for real people in the real world. Your inner goddess will thank you, as will the Adonis in him.

Sensual Massage

There's nothing more intimate that the touch of your lover. Enjoy massaging each other, consider it foreplay. Set the mood by lighting candles, putting on soft music and grabbing a bottle of lotion or oil. There are lots of aromatherapy lotions available. KY Brand also has several massaging oils, vaginal moisturizers, lubricants, and climax enhancers.

FOR HER
One way to add an extra special touch after awarding him with a massage is to finish by giving him a handjob. If you've never given a handjob ask him to stroke himself with your hand on the outside of his hands. Take note of the speed and pressure he uses, and then immolate his actions. If you begin to get tired switch hands, or use both hands to make it a little easier for you.

FOR HIM
Remember, a relaxed woman will have more energy and desire for other activities, namely sexing you up. As a special treat for her, you may consider giving her a full body massage that doesn't lead to sex. Take a raincheck on the sex, but know its coming; she'll be grateful you put her needs first.

Rub a Dub in the Tub

One of the most sensual acts between lovers is taking a bath together. As simple as hot water and hot bodies, or go all out with bubbles, candles, and soft music. If you want to take the experience further, make love in the bath.

FOR HER
The easiest way to make love in the tub is for the female to straddle her husband. Once you start riding him, the water can overflow so keep in mind the water level before you begin. Be prepared to let some of the water out to keep the floor dry.

FOR HIM
Another position for tub loving is to have your wife on her hands and knees and do it doggie style. You can also have her stand in the tub, lean down and hold onto the side then take her from behind. *Safety Note: Because the water and soap may be slippery, be very careful not to thrust too hard which may cause her to lose her balance.*

Mirror, Mirror

Make love in front of the mirror. Watch as your lover ravishes you.

FOR HER
Men are visual. They love to look at your body while you make love. Let him indulge by standing in front of the mirror as he takes you.

FOR HIM
Women are resistant to the mirror. They may be self-conscience about their bodies and all the movement that comes from making love. Reassure her that you love the way she looks, especially when you're making love.

Email Me

Foreplay doesn't have to start five minutes before you get busy. Begin foreplay by sending emails or text messages to each other. Let your lover know you are thinking of them in a sexual way. Drop hints about what you'll do to each other when you are together again. You can also use emails to stay connected to your spouse. Imagine how great it will feel when you open your mailbox and know that your spouse is thinking of you. That, in and of itself, is a subtle form of foreplay.

FOR HER
Send short emails or text with simple phrases describing your husband's favorite body part. This will entice him and make him think of you all day long.

FOR HIM
When you send her an email or text remind her how much she means to you. Let her know what you'd like to do to her later. Then, do it!

Shave Me

FOR HER
Shave your pussy or let him shave you. Keep in mind, when the hair grows back it itches like crazy. You can cut down on this itching by keeping yourself shaved or by shaving just the hair on the labia. It can be very sexual to have your husband shave you. This is a testament to trust in your relationship. You can also try waxing. It is painful so take two ibuprofen thirty minutes before your appointment. *Safety Note: Be careful with a razor around your clitoris. Make sure to use a new razor and plenty of shaving cream. You may want to use scissors to shorten the hair before you begin to shave.*

FOR HIM
Allow her to shave your face. Make sure to give her plenty of instruction so she doesn't cut you. She will be nervous, so be patient and kind with your instruction. You want this to be romantic and part of foreplay.

Why not reciprocate the hair free zone by shaving your testicles and pubic hair for her? If you like the look, have her shave you next time. Blowjobs are much more fun when she isn't worrying about tiny hairs getting stuck in her throat.

Silky Hair

WASHING
This can be very intimate and sensual. Most people love to have their head massaged and scratched. As you are washing your lover's hair, massage their scalp and scratch their head.

BRAIDING
Christen braids Ana's hair to keep it out of the way. Teach your husband to braid your hair. You can also pull it into a ponytail. That works great to give him something to hold onto while he's driving himself into you.

PULLING
Many men and women enjoy having their hair pulled during intercourse. Just remember your scalp has millions of nerve endings, it only takes a gentle tug to get the desired effect. Pull too hard and you cause more pain than pleasure.

TWISTING
Men love to twist/fist their hand in your hair. Give him a chance to twist your hair while he forces you to give him a blowjob.

Shower Sex

Take a shower together and let your lover wash your body. To add a special touch, shower in the dark. Your sense of touch will be heightened.

FOR HER
Men don't usually use bath sponges, but women know how wonderfully relaxing they can be. Use a bath sponge while you wash his body, nice and slow.

FOR HIM
When your body is soapy, rub against her; who says you can't get a little dirty in the shower. Hot water streaming down your bodies can be very titillating. *Safety Note: If you decide to make love in the shower, remember the floor will be very slippery. Use caution.*

Making Out

Making out is a lost art. No one makes out anymore. Of course, who has the time? You have to make time for making out. It's the ultimate foreplay. The next time you're watching TV, make out like you were teenagers. Kiss, fondle, get hot, but do not go all the way. Or do go all the way, but only after at least fifteen minutes of making out.

FOR HER
A fun way to make out is to give your husband a blowjob during commercial breaks. When your program resumes, stop the blowjob until the next commercial break.

FOR HIM
Remember going around the bases in high school. Here's your chance for the major leagues. Round the bases with your lady, but do not go for the homeroom. If you do knock one out of the park, give her at least fifteen minutes of making out before you slide home.

Satin Sheets

Satin sheets scream sex. The feel of satin against your skin brings to mind the sensual feelings of romance. You can enjoy satin sheets every night or only on special occasions. Buy a set and use them for special nights. You can also put them on the morning of a planned hot night of sex. Each time you walk past them you'll anticipate the fun you'll be having later. Red and black are my favorites.

Mutual Masturbation

This is lots of fun, but can be intimidating. Take your time, dim the lights, have a glass of wine and show each other what feels good.

FOR HER
Nothing will get your man hotter than watching you masturbate. If you are uncomfortable you can ask him to go first; or you can go at the same time. You can also wear a blindfold; sometimes this helps to ease anxiety. Remember, men are visual, so the sight of his lover pleasuring herself will be a huge turn-on.

FOR HIM
When you masturbate for your wife, show her the way you like to be touched. She can incorporate special touches during oral sex and handjobs.

Pin Me Down

A simple way to be dominated is to be restrained during intercourse. Your husband can pin you down and have his way with you or you can turn the tables and pin him down. Pick up any Cosmo magazine and you'll see the number one thing men want is for their women to take charge in the bedroom more often. Now's your chance to take him and do all kinds of naughty things.

FOR HER
When you sit riding him, hold his arms down so that he is under your complete control.

FOR HIM
Restrain her by simply holding her wrists, hands, or arms as you take her. You can also hold her hands above her head when you're inside her.

Taste Me

Why is it that tasting our own juices is so freaking hot? Maybe because it seems a little taboo.

FOR HER
When you masturbate have him lick your fingers clean when you're finished. After you've gone down on him and he comes in your mouth, make sure to kiss him. It can be very erotic to share such an intimate act.

FOR HIM
When was the last time your fingered your woman? Add this act to your foreplay. When you two are both hot and bothered and your fingers are covered with her excitement, have her lick your fingers clean. Don't be afraid to taste your own come. She does it, if it's good enough for her, its good enough for you.

Undress Me

When you take clothes off your spouse, you are in control. This simple act can be very powerful.

FOR HER
After a long day of work, seduce your man by undressing him. Add sexual tension by whispering how good he looks under his working man clothes. Above all else, take your time. Excruciatingly slow clothes removal can lead to incredibly hot lovemaking.

FOR HIM
Show your wife how much she excites you by undressing her. With each piece of clothing that drops to the floor, lick the exposed skin. It's a great way to get her wet, in all the right places.

Cover My Eyes

Take away your sense of sight and all other senses are heightened. A great way to be a submissive is to give yourself over without seeing what is happening around you. How hot is that? Suggestions: blindfold, a tie, a scarf, a pillow (cover just eyes, not entire face), a pillow case over the head.
(Safety Note: Be extremely careful covering your lover's mouth/nose. Make sure he/she can always say the Safeword and that you can hear the Safeword.)

Side Note: Once my husband shoved me into our closet and put a pillowcase over my head. I didn't realize I was claustrophobic, but it freaked me the hell out. So, be prepared, you never know how someone will react, even if you've discussed the game play beforehand.

FOR HER
When you're blindfolded, enjoy the touches of your lover. Listening to music with ear buds, as Ana did, can add to the sensual atmosphere.

FOR HIM
Allow your wife to blindfold you, then enjoy not knowing what's coming next.

Kissing

Kiss freely, Kiss frequently

When you're driving in your car, kiss your lover's hand. This act of affection connects you.

Take advantage of mistletoe during the holiday season. Don't miss every opportunity to smooch a little when you stand under it.

French kiss AT LEAST once a day. Make it a priority. Not a peck on the cheek, but tongue lashing mouth-on-mouth assaults.

Kiss goodnight. Every night.

Every time you leave each other's company; kiss goodbye.

Kiss for no reason. Just KISS.

ROUGHIN' IT

The second part of the book focuses on mixing things up and getting down and dirty. The ideas in this section may push you a little outside your comfort zone, but give them a try. You may be surprised to find you actually enjoy being naughty.

Safeword

Anytime you participate in sex games you need to
create a Safeword prior to play and ALWAYS use the
Safeword if you feel uncomfortable or are in pain;
not pleasurable pain, but painful pain.

Try to use the same Safeword every time you
participate in kinky sex. This way when you get all
worked up, it will be easier to remember.

Quite common are the words: Red, Yellow, Green.
Red means stop IMMEDIATELY. Yellow means you
are almost at your threshold of pain tolerance. Green
means everything is okay; I love what you're doing.
Oftentimes, the dominant will say 'green' as a way of
checking on their partner's pleasure. (It's a little
sexier to say 'green', than to ask, Are you okay? Does
this feel good? Should I keep going?)

If you or your spouse ever disrespects the Safeword,
then you should NEVER play rough again. You can't
enjoy yourself if you are worried that he/she won't
stop when things get too scary or painful. Please
respect your partner.

Of Great Importance: Safesign
If your submissive has something in her mouth and
can't speak, you need to develop signs to
communicate that play needs to stop. A few

examples are: holding something in your hand and when play gets too rough dropping it. You could also tap your partner on the head 3 times or slap the floor 3 times.

Ripping Panties

FOR HER
If you want your husband to turn into a wild animal, give him permission to rip your clothes off. You can take an old t-shirt or older bra/underwear and have him unleash the beast within. Note you will need to start the tear prior to his wild behavior. Remember you will be unleashing the animal in him, be prepared for animalistic loving to follow!

FOR HIM
Ripping off your wife's underwear can bring out the animal in you. Take note it can bruise her because although it is done easily enough in the movies, in real life material doesn't tear without some preliminary work. Prior to ravaging your wife, you need to cut a slit along the seam so that it will be easier to rip apart. Of course, make sure you have her permission before you start cutting her underwear.

Vehicle Loving

Think back to your high school days when you didn't have the money or a place to make love. You resorted to the backside of your vehicle. Why not relive those glory days by going parking.

FOR HER
Based on the type of vehicle you have, you straddling your husband is fairly easy to accomplish in cars or trucks. If you can push the front seat down and get onto all fours, you can have him take you from behind. This can take some practice and flexibility, but its lots of fun.

FOR HIM
You can also have her lie over the hood and take her from behind. *Safety Note: The hood of the car might be hot, so you may need to wait a while before you start making whoopee splayed across the hood. Making out in the front seat for about ten minutes will give you time to heat her up while your car cools down.*

Hickies

Hickies are generally left for the adolescent who has no self-control. But they can be sexy and fun as hell to give and get. If you're interested in reliving your glory days and test your hicky giving/getting ability, you may consider putting them in areas hidden by clothing. Plus, it's extra fun when you know what's hiding under your clothing. Every time you see it, it will remind you of how you got it.

Against the Wall

You can fuck against any wall in the house. Just make sure no one is home!

FOR HER
Stand with your back against the wall and have your husband enter you, then put your legs together, the friction can be exhilarating. The friction causes him to rub against your clitoris and orgasm is much easier.

FOR HIM
You can have her stand facing the wall with her arms to the side (looks like a cop is searching you) and take her from behind. You can also have her bend at the waist and take her while slapping her ass with each thrust.

Stairway to Heaven

If you have stairs in your home, consider yourself lucky. It's one of the sexist architectural design elements in a house.

FOR HER
The easiest way to make love on the stairs is to get on all fours and have him take you from behind. *Safety Note: Be careful of carpet burn. With all the friction, your knees can burn. You may want to put a pillow under them.*

FOR HIM
Another fun way to have sex on stairs is to have your wife lie back on the stairs then put her foot against the wall and the other foot against the stair railing. She can thrust upward thanks to the resistance of the wall/railing. *Safety Note: For her, put a pillow to make sure her butt doesn't get carpet burn.*

Sex Toys

Oh the fun that can be had with sex toys. There are so many varieties available. It can be sexy and exciting trying out things you've never done before. *Safety Note: Make sure to clean your toys after each playtime. You can put condoms over vibrators and dildos to make cleaning easier.*

FOR HER
Don't be afraid to try toys that make you a little nervous. Just remember your Safeword. Getting out of your comfort level usually brings the greatest sexual pleasure.

FOR HIM
Don't be afraid to let her use her toys on you. It's very manly to be pleasured by your wife. She plays with the equipment therefore she knows some of the best ways to use it. Let loose and have a blast.

A FEW TO TRY:
Dildo
Vibrator
Cock Ring
Flavored Condoms
Flavored Lube
*Triple Stimulator (this is my favorite). It's a dildo with a cock ring attached and a vibrator. Your husband puts the cock ring on his penis and uses the dildo so that you can be double penetrated while the

vibrator rubs your clitoris. You two can decide if the vibrator will go in your anus or your pussy. The dildo is flexible which means g-spot stimulating. Double penetration with the love of your life. Hell Yeah!

Woman on Top

Is he always in control? It's her turn now. Woman on top gives her complete control: speed and depth are her choice.

FOR HER
Ride him hard, ride him fast, ride him slow. It's your choice. Woman on top is an easy way to orgasm because you control the speed and the depth. You can easily rub your clit over his pubic bone almost guaranteeing an orgasm. Make sure and twist around so that his cock can rub different areas inside your vagina.

FOR HIM
Give her a hand by holding her hips and helping her ride you. You can also help out by twisting and pinching her nipples as she rides you. If you put your knees up she can lean back and you can rub her clit while she grinds against you.

Spank Me

When you think of kinky sex, one of the first things people think about is spanking. Guys like to get spanked as much as women do. Talk to your spouse and see if spanking is something he/she wants. Sometimes the sound is hotter than the slap. The sound of slapping someone can be an extreme turn-on. Spanking can be used for sexual pleasure or as punishment when your partner disobeys you. You can use your hand for gentle swats and work your way to more intentional pain infliction: wooden spoon, plastic spatula, ping pong paddle, belt, flip flop, hairbrush, ruler, book, folded magazine or newspaper.

FOR HER
Men like to be spanked as much as women. Don't forget to discuss it with your husband and remember to respect the Safeword. You can swat him while you do it missionary or when he takes you against the wall while you wrap your legs around him.

FOR HIM
Typically men like to spank women when they're going at it doggie style. If she has disobeyed you, spank her before you pleasure her. Bend her over your knees and teach her who the real boss is. Remember if she uses the Safeword, you must respect that and STOP immediately.

Handcuffs

Handcuffs are a necessity for any kinky sex kit. You never know how much pain your body can handle and how much you might enjoy it until the handcuffs come out. They come in many styles: plain metal, leather, pink fur, or black vinyl and others. Your pick.

FOR HER
Handcuffs are fun, but can bite your skin. Be prepared with ointment afterward. Play cop and criminal and let him use his cuffs to 'take you in'.

FOR HIM
While she's handcuffed finger her until she begs you to stop or begs you to replace your finger with something a bit more substantial.

Fuzzy Fur

In the novel, the first time Christina ties Ana up, he uses a furry glove to caress her body. How sensual is that? You can do the same with or without a furry glove. You can use a stuffed animal or a piece of fur from an arts & crafts store. You can use a feather duster (new, of course), or a strip of satin.

Take your time; do not rush through foreplay. It's sensual to both partners and a great way to get everyone warmed up.

KINKY FUCKERY

The third part of *Fifty Shades of Grey for Couples*
pulls out all the stops. This is where you separate the
dom from the sub. Hey, just go for it: kinky play
every night! My favorite extreme website is: Extreme
Restraints
www.extremerestraints.com

Sir or Mistress

The first step to kinky fuckery is how you address your partner. Demand respect by requiring a subordinate to address you by Sir or Mistress. It's the first sign you are in the dominant position. By responding with Sir or Mistress you show your lover you are willing to turn over your power, which is the ultimate aphrodisiac. So, let lose, let go and give it up!

FOR HER
Be prepared for whatever your Master asks of you. Always address your Master with Sir. It's not only respectful, it's a turn-on.

FOR HIM
When you decide to allow your wife to dominate you, remember to address her as Mistress. This will help you to stay submissive and give her the dominant power in your love play. Understand, Sir?

Anal Plug (Butt Plug)

Butt Plug and Anal Plug are terms used interchangeably. An anal plug is a sexual toy inserted in the anus for sexual gratification. It can be used by males or females. It tends to be shorter than rubber dildos. It has a flanged end which prevents it from going in too deep which can damage your colon. They also come with vibrators inside so your partner can turn the vibrator on while it's inserted in your rectum for additional stimulation. Oftentimes, butt plugs are foreplay for anal sex. They tend to stretch and relax your sphincter muscles in preparation for a penis. *Safety Note: Always clean your sex toys after use with warm soap and water. Never use a sex toy in your anus and vagina during the same lovemaking session. The rectum has bacteria that can cause illness.*

FOR HER

If you've never used a butt plug, start slowly and use lots of lubrication. You can leave the butt plug in for extra stimulation as your husband fucks you. *If you've used them before and are relatively comfortable, try the butt plugs that have vibrators inside them for a little extra kink.*

FOR HIM

Don't be afraid of the butt plug for your own sexual pleasure. Have your wife lube your rectum and slowly insert a butt plug. For extra boldness, you too can try the vibrating butt plugs.

Anal Beads

Anal beads are sex toys used for sexual pleasure. They consist of several balls attached in a series. You insert the beads into the anus and remove them at orgasm. By pulling the beads out either quickly or slowly during your orgasm, you may reach new levels of pleasure you've never experienced before. Make sure to use plenty of lubricant before inserting the anal beads.

Safety Note: Many anal beads come with a string that can be difficult to clean properly. You can insert them into a condom to keep them sanitary. It's best not to share anal beads between partners without thoroughly cleaning them. It's recommended to purchase anal beads that are a continuous piece of silicone. If you purchased anal beads with the string, always count the beads after anal play. The string could break during 'rough play' and a ball could become lodged or left in the rectum.

FOR HER

Have him tell you when his orgasm begins and slowly pull the anal beads out to enhance his orgasm. Try pulling them slowly one time, next time pull quicker.

FOR HIM

As you give her oral sex and she reaches orgasm, pull the anal beads out enhancing her orgasm. Try different speeds until you find the one that gives her the greatest pleasure.

Nipple Clamps

Nipple clamps are clips that are clamped onto your nipples. They can be used by men or women, most frequently women. Nipple clamps restrict blood flow which causes pain/pleasure. There are many different types available. Some are adjustable so you can change the pressure being applied. You can apply nipple clamps onto one breast or both. It is highly erotic to see nipple clamps on both nipples with a chain hanging between them. Some Masters enjoy tugging on the chain causing pleasurable ripples of pain. Before placing a nipple clamp make sure you prepare your nipple. Get it nice and hard, tease it, pinch it. Remember the more skin you pinch into the clamp the less pressure, the smaller the area the more pressure will be applied.

Safety Note: If you pinch just the tip of the nipple you are more likely to damage your nipple causing severe pain. Again, pinch as much skin as possible when you are first learning to play. This will help prevent damage and you'll have more fun.

Safety Note II: It's recommended they stay on no longer than 10 to 15 minutes. You'll want to keep in mind nipple clamps hurt more when you take them off as the blood rushes back to the erect nipple.

Genital Clamps

Genital clamps are much like nipple clamps. They are used to restrict blood flood to your genitals, both male and female. This type of kinky fuckery is not for the fate of heart. It can be pleasurable, but extremely painful.

Safety Note: Keep a close eye on skin color changes. Restricting blood flow for too long can cause permanent damage. Also remember certain areas of the skin are too thin and sensitive for clamps (think inner labia for a woman).

FOR BOTH
Pick up a clamp and pinch a lot of skin and see how you enjoy the feeling.

Wartenberg Pinwheel

A Wartenberg pinwheel is an instrument used for nerve stimulation. It's a rolling pinwheel that has sharp points. You roll the pinwheel over different parts of your lover's body to give them intense pleasure. Areas of the body that you wouldn't think are sensitive to this stimulation can be discovered as a couple. *Safety Note: Read the directions carefully to avoid puncturing the skin. The points are generally not sharp enough to damage the skin unless you apply excessive pressure. Remember to respect the Safeword.*

FOR HER
Run the pinwheel along his chest and neck. A man's neck is full of nerve endings. Have fun, find his favorite spot.

FOR HIM
Have her lie on her stomach and roll the pinwheel along the back of her legs. This area can be extremely sensitive, especially behind her knees. You can also run it along the sole of her feet (this might be ticklish, so be prepared).

Ball Gag

Ball gags are part of bondage play and are perfect for fulfilling your dom/sub fantasies. Use ball gags as punishment for speaking without permission or as a way to muffle screams of pain or sounds of pleasure. Ball gags come in a range of styles and collars. Most definitely discuss your Safesign before you insert a ball gag in his/her mouth. You'll need a signal in case play gets too rough. (See Safeword)

FOR HER
Now, you can control him. Put a ball gag in his mouth. Enough said.

FOR HIM
You know she talks constantly. Finally, a way to shut her up: slip a ball gag in her mouth.

Spreader Bar

A spreader bar is usually adjustable and used with wrist or ankle restraints to keep your lover positioned just for you. Keep the one you're dominating restrained and spread as far as you like. Try different positions to keep your submissive right where you want them, positioned for pleasure.

Riding Crop

Getting punished with a riding crop is one of the more painful ways to bring pleasure. Start slowly so that you can judge marks that may be left on your lover's body. Riding crops are perfect for beginning domination or as fantasy play between consenting adults.

FOR HER
When you want to dominate him, use your riding crop to make him do exactly what you desire.

FOR HIM
Blindfold your lover, then trace her body with the crop before you punish her with a good old-fashioned spanking.

Period Sex

This is one of the more taboo forms of sex. Some women love it, some hate it. Some men enjoy it, others think it's gross. Always use a condom to prevent infections. Discuss this with your lover. It's preferable in the shower or tub. If you decide to have period sex on your bed, place a dark towel under you.

FOR HER
If you get super horny while on your period, you don't have to wait until it's over to enjoy sex. Have your spouse use a condom and communicate constantly while you're enjoying each other.

FOR HIM
If your wife drives you so crazy that you can't wait until she's finished with her cycle, then enjoy period sex. Missionary position seems to be the most pleasurable for women during their period. Other positions tend to have your penis jabbing ovaries and causing discomfort. Discuss this with your lover.

Ben Wa Balls

Christian loved for Ana to wear these and Ana was excited to wear them. These are marble sized balls that are inserted in the vagina. They are generally used for sexual stimulation and can also be used to strengthen your Kegel muscles. To strengthen your Kegels pretend you are urinating, then stop the flow. Do these thirty times three times a day. Stronger Kegel muscles greatly enhance your orgasm. Ben Wa balls come in different sizes and weights, so do research before you purchase them.

FOR HER
Practice your Kegels using Ben Wa balls and Kegel exercises. You'll be glad you did, as will he, because you can squeeze his penis while he's inside you.

FOR HIM
Have her wear them to dinner and the movies. Only you and her know what dirty thing she's doing. When you get back home, she'll be more than ready to be taken.

Tied Up

How many times did Christian tie Ana up? I lost count. But, it sure made me want to be tied and taken. There are lots of common items that can be used to tie your lover up: scarf, tie, pantyhose, leggings, belt, rope, yarn, shoestrings, belt of a robe.

FOR HER
Tie him up spread eagle on your bed. Use ice to trace a path along his body or tickle him with a feather. To really keep him guessing, blindfold him. With him tied, you can tease him, walk away make him wait five minutes or so, then go back to pleasing him. Do this several times. He'll be putty in your hands.

FOR HIM
Tie her face down on the bed spread eagle then have your way with her backside (with her permission). Explore her body with your tongue. Don't stop until she begs you to.

Vibrators

Vibrators come in many shapes, sizes, and varieties. There are those you wear, those that fit conveniently into a pair of panties, those shaped like a penis, and so many more. If you don't have one, pick one out together. If you have one but only use it for masturbation, pull it out during lovemaking. There are lots of fun ways to use it with your spouse.

FOR HER
Use a vibrator to play with his testicles. With his permission, insert the vibrator into his anus; use plenty of lube and a condom. If he is unsure about this, ease into it. First time just rub the vibrator around the rim of his rectum. Next time use your finger to loosen him up, then insert an inch of the vibrator. Keeping working until he can take the entire length.

FOR HIM
With a condom on, you can insert the vibrator in her ass while you take her doggie style, or any position.

Married Sex: Erotica for Couples

Looking to have a night of passion with the one you've vowed to have and to hold? Hoping to rekindle sex and intimacy in your relationship? Seduce your lover with these fantasies that will ignite your fire and scorch your sheets. In *Married Sex: Erotica for Couples*, eight erotic stories combine lust and love with tales of wanton behavior and sexual explorations sure to spark an inferno.

These enticing fantasies include spanking, voyeurism, couple swapping, three-ways, group sex and sensual adventures that will challenge couples to reach new heights of sexual satisfaction.

Now available for Kindle and Amazon CreateSpace

Sizzling Hot Sex Tips

Tried and true ways to get your lover hot and bothered, and a few new ones to try. Work your way through the entire list.

Chocolate – drizzle chocolate on each other and lick it off.

Tender caress – touching can be very erotic. Explore the contours of your lover's body with your fingers and fingertips.

Minty mouth – pop a peppermint before you go down on your lover.

Sexy MadLibs – fill in the blank: I want to _____ your _____. (verb/body part)

Go to a sex toy store together and BUY something fun.

Naked breakfast in bed.

Pearl necklace – use flavored lube to wrap pearls around his member before going down on him.

Sex slave – be a slave to love for one night.

Island Paradise – transform your bedroom into a tropical oasis with exotic flowers, Hawaiian music, and flower leis, then make love in paradise.

Hidden quickie – sneak into the bathroom and write an invitation for a quickie on the mirror, when it steams up, your message will appear.

Rent an adult movie and watch it together.

Treasure trail, leave a path of clothes to the bedroom.

Strip poker.

Sticky sex – write sexy notes on sticky notes and leave them for your lover to find.

Tickle me with a feather.

Tattoo – hunt and find. Buy a temporary tattoo and hide it somewhere on your body then have your lover try to find it.

Take sexy photos of each other.

Video tape your lovemaking, and then watch it together.

Phone sex using your cell phones; even if you're in the same house. You go to one room, your spouse go to the other.

Read erotic story aloud. (check out my Erotica for Couples collection)

Write part of erotic story together. You write one chapter then have your partner write the next chapter.

Call your spouse at work and talk dirty to them.

Oral sex while driving.

Go commando. (no underwear)

During missionary put your legs on his shoulder and a pillow under your butt.

Give him a hand job in the movie theater.

When riding reverse cowgirl, lean down and grab his ankles.

Naked twister.

Dirty dance.

Cook naked wearing nothing but an apron and stilettos. (nothing that splatters)

Eat naked.

Clean naked.

Sex board game. Buy an adult board game and play together.

Go to bar and get picked up by a stranger (your spouse).

Suck her toes.

Sex with your heels on.

Go to an adult toy shop and BUY something.

Whip cream bikini.

Sleeping bag sex.

Sexy lingerie for him and her.

Truth or dare. (A fun way to get to know your lover is to play this while driving, focusing more on the truth part. You can learn a whole lot about your significant other).

Dry hump on the sofa during a movie.

Use ice to seduce your lover.

Dirty talk. Don't be afraid to SCREAM. Men love to hear their woman scream with pleasure.

69 side by side or with him on top. Hang your head off the bed so that he can drive his cock deeper into your mouth.

Bite her, nibble her, claw him.

Use a clear shower curtain so that your lover can watch your shower.

Wear a thong.

Go braless.

Pull your underwear to the side and have him take you. The urgency is hot!

Suck fast, lick slow.

Wake him up with a morning BJ.

As soon as he walks in, push him against the wall and take him.

Vow to have sex in one form or another for seven days straight.

Put your lacy undies in his pants pocket as an all day reminder of you.

Wear knee high boots, a trench coat, a smile, and nothing else.

Skype sex.

On the way home, the closer you get, move your hand closer to his package, then when you get there, and give him a hand job.

Bend over the sink and let him take you from behind, watching in the mirror.

When he comes home, make sure you're naked and spread eagle on the bed.

Put condom on using your mouth. (Place the condom with the tip against the roof of your mouth; use your teeth to hold it in place the lower your mouth onto his cock. Use your tongue to roll it down. It might take some practice so buy some flavored condoms. If you don't need condoms for protection, it can still be fun to play with them).

Have sex where you switch positions at least 5 times.

Share sexual fantasies; try to make one come true.

Role play. Doctor/Patient, Nurse/Doctor, Nurse/Patient, College Professor/Student, Policeman/Law-Breaking Citizen, Housewife/Handyman, Boss/Secretary, Postman/Lonely Housewife, Stripper/Horny Customer, Lingerie Model/Horny Customer, Airline Steward/Passenger, Drill Sergeant/Private, any others you'd like to try. Be creative!

Go on an old fashioned date. Go to the front door and pick her up.

Rent a hotel that has a Jacuzzi tub and let the jets stimulate you to orgasm while he watches. He can assist by pinching/twisting your nipples or kissing your neck or whatever your sexual trigger is.

With his permission, during oral insert a finger in his anus. *you can buy finger covers at the medical supply section of a drugstore if you're a little squeamish.

Use the internet and find the nearest drive-in movie theater, go there and make out during the movie. If the movie is boring, go all the way in the backseat.

Kiss, lick and caress every inch of her/his body.

Use your feet to masturbate him (a foot job).

Give him a 30 minute blowjob: slow, wet, and thorough.

Perform oral sex on her until she orgasms three times.

Sofa Loving – she puts her knees on seat of sofa, lean over the headrest while he stands behind you and takes you.

Sofa Loving II – he sits on sofa, you stand on sofa straddling him, place your knees on either side of his head then lower yourself so that he can perform orally.

Have him sex you up with a dildo while he kneels near your mouth while you suck him.

Tied Up

Ryan walked in the door and dropped his stuff on the counter. He'd suffered a hard day when nothing went right, and felt completely drained. Walking into the bedroom, he thought about lying down and taking a nap, but figured if he did that he'd wake up then probably have trouble going to sleep later. Instead, he went into the bathroom. Looking at the jacuzzi tub he thought for a second about soaking, but ditched the idea for a simple hot shower. He'd just stripped naked when he heard the garage door open. He stepped into the steaming water, and stood there, letting it relax his aching muscles and pound his neck, relieving the tension. The water trickled over his package, giving him a slight stimulation, causing him to relax even more. The door burst open as Amy, his wife, hurried in, quickly slamming the door shut, and snapping at him, "I hope you haven't used all the hot water."

He quelled the smart-assed comment that came to his lips and sighed. It looked like they'd both had a bad day.

"Where are the girls?" He asked.

"Softball," was all she said. She then went on to explain the girls were both having a sleepover with friends after softball practice and it would be just the two of them for dinner.

"How was your day?" Ryan asked.

Amy related that she'd a terrible day. She was a teacher, and her students had acted like little monsters, with the principal observing her class. She'd been a nervous wreck and had referred several students to detention, which then caused them to leave and call their parents to whine. After that, those parents had called the school to complain. She shared this as she began stripping her clothes off. His cock twitched as she leaned forward, allowing her bra to fall free of her full breasts, rubbing where the straps had left marks on her skin. Ryan's rod rose a bit, as she unconsciously cupped her tits massaging the ripe flesh, then slipped her hand into the waistband of her panties. She was turned slightly, but glancing past her in the mirror, he could see the material as it slipped into her ass crack. He stood, frozen, watching her peel the thin cotton from her pale skin, mesmerized as she pulled the cloth from her cleft exposing her thick hairy bush. She noticed him staring.

She sighed, then in a contemptuous voice said, "Control yourself stud, I'm not in the mood."

Ryan replied, "Maybe it's just what you need."

She ignored him and stepped into the shower, taking the soap from him. "I want a hot shower, a good book, and a relaxing evening on the sofa."

Amy appeared to be ignoring his semi-erect cock. He rubbed her ass as his cock grew harder. She gave an exasperated exhale and started soaping her body, only adding to his predicament of a semi-hard dick feeling neglected. He got the message and stepped

back, watching her wash as his abandoned dick
bounced with every heartbeat. He rolled his eyes as
she washed her thatch of fur, teasing him in an
almost painfully seductive way. She glimpsed him
standing there, hard and ready.

Finally she mumbled, "Maybe later."

A white bolt of anger shot through his chest, but
Ryan said nothing and started to step out.

Amy mouthed, "What's wrong? Giving up so easily?"
He looked at her, then stepped forward only to hear
her say, "Not now, maybe later!"

He'd suffered enough snotty comments, and took
swift action, grabbing her and smashing his lips hard
over hers. She dropped the soap as he forced her
into the wall. His arms enclosed her as she wrestled
against him.

"Get off me," she snarled, as he broke the forceful
kiss.

She got an arm loose, but Ryan twisted it behind her
back, spinning her around his half-hard dick swinging
from side-to-side. He secured her other arm and held
her tight, pressing her hands together, securing her
thumbs in his left hand, and freeing his right. He
nudged the faucet, turning the water off. Amy
resisted, kicking at him. Ryan silently pushed her out
of the shower, through the bathroom, and into the
bedroom. They dripped water everywhere, but he
didn't care. Frustration and other negative emotions
bled away; as he brought the contemptuous woman
he'd married to heel. She was acting like a haughty

little *not now I've got a headache* prima donna.
Ryan was about to show her who was boss. She'd
teased him on purpose, and now she'd pay the price.
He grabbed a scarf from her dresser drawer and
quickly tied her hands behind her back. Shoving her
face down on the bed, he grabbed another scarf and
tied her left foot to the bedpost before tying her
right foot to the other. Collecting a final scarf, Ryan
straddled her ass and untied her hands. The whole
time she fought and twisted, giving him a nice ride as
her jiggling butt squeezed his dick between her pale,
round moons.

Leaning his weight on her, listening to her foul
cursing and heavy breathing, he tied her hands over
her head, finally tying the scarf to the headboard and
ensuring her hands were secure. Ryan stepped back
to admire his handiwork. Amy glared at him, and the
things she threatened him with would have made his
nuts draw up, if they didn't excite him so much.

His angry conquest was so hot; he couldn't imagine
how he'd been so lucky to have snagged her. He
slapped her voluptuous ass, watching the flesh turn
an angry red. He grabbed a handful, squeezing and
rubbing, kneading the flesh of her fine ass until his
cock leaked fluid, leaving a clear drop on her hip
where it rested. Ryan swiped it up with his finger,
generously rubbing it over her luscious lips. When
she thought he wasn't watching, she secretly licked
her lips, tasting the salty sweet pre-cum.

"Gotcha!" Ryan said triumphantly, "I saw that."

"Fuck you!" She spit back. He laughed as she fought

against the bonds, and then Ryan eased his dick toward her face as she threatened, "I'll bite it. I swear to you. I'll bite it off."

Ryan straddled her back, grabbing her hair firmly, twisting her face toward him. Instead of thrusting toward her tight lips and clenched teeth, he rubbed his cock on her cheek, across her nose and over her face; her hair tickling his balls. He was careful to avoid her mouth. His other hand gripped a handful of pale ass flesh as he thrust his pelvis forward, keeping control of her by her hair. Ryan released her ass, and leaning forward he took his pulsating cock and slapped her face with it. Carefully, he popped her on the face, milking his dick until a large clear drop of pre-cum emerged. He smeared it on her face, right at the corner of her mouth, careful to make sure she couldn't make good on her promise to bite him. He stood up as she licked his cream from her cheek with her talented tongue.

She writhed against her bonds, her green eyes glowing. "So much fire," he spit at her. "Tonight it won't go to waste."

Amy was so different from the tense woman who'd walked into the shower just a few minutes earlier. Her heart pounded, her breathing was heavy, and a thin sheen of sweat had replaced the water from the shower. Ryan even felt different from the tired, beat person who'd come home after a day where everything went wrong. They both knew what it was, too. Ryan and Amy both needed this release, and the transformation had been natural, as had everything in their love life.

They'd come home beaten down by the world, and had slipped away into their own place away from it all; to a world where the emotions they felt for each other, and the secret desires they both had, came true. It could have just as easily been him tied up there, with her exercising control. Fortunately, it was her day to be taken. Ryan went to the kitchen, grabbed a beer, and headed back toward the bedroom. Leaning on the doorjamb sipping the cold brew, he watched his wife struggle. His cock hung half-hard as he let the anticipation grow. Finally, he shut the door and locked it.

First, Ryan took down the small box from the closet that held the sex toys they hid from the kids. He sat it on the dresser and selected a bottle of lubricant, then took a towel from the bathroom, forcing it under her writhing body. She almost got him with a knee as he adjusted the towel. He vehemently told her, "That'll cost you."

He took the thick black vibrator and a condom from the box. At that moment, he was glad she made them use condoms to keep their toys clean; no wasted time cleaning the Bushmaster, her favorite toy. He rolled the condom over the vibrator, tying the rubber securely. As he spread the lube over the toy dick, she warned him again to stay away from her. Of course, Ryan ignored her; straddling her with his ass toward her head, looking down at the prize of her jiggling butt.

Ryan trailed the vibrator along Amy's ass crack, gently probing, anxious to slip it inside; knowing she was equally anxious to get fucked by it. He had to make her wait a little longer, and make her suffer for the nasty comments about biting his dick. He turned the toy on; rubbing it slowly along her ass down to her upper thighs, he listened intently for the moans he knew would soon be escaping her. He began to probe her pussy lips as she unintentionally spread her legs, giving him full access. Ryan rubbed alongside her pussy touching her clit with the vibrating toy, leaving it in place for several seconds; knowing the intense vibrations would be just what she needed.

"You ready to be good? Or do I need to punish you a little more for being bad?"

"Fuck you!"

"Okay, you asked for it." He swatted her ass, causing it to wiggle and turn pink. She whimpered, which of course encouraged him to do it again. Ryan smacked her ass a little harder. One, two, three swats, leaving a crimson-red handprint.

"I said fuck you and I mean it! Fuck you. Now untie me, I don't want to play."

"You don't want to play? Let's see if you're lying." He slipped his hand between her thighs to test her pussy lips, anxious to see if she was as wet as he hoped she was. Sure enough, her cunt drenched his fingers.

"Seems to me, you're more than ready to play. Your pussy is soaking wet, even wet the towel a little; a clear sign you're enjoying getting your ass spanked." Ryan leaned down beside her ear and whispered tenderly, "If you really don't want to play, just say the safe word and I'll stop."

"Fuck you. I don't need you to get me off; I'm perfectly capable of doing that myself."

"Well, we'll see about that later. Right now, I'm having fun, and I'm not ready to stop."

Her loving husband took the vibrator and began to slide it in and out of her wanton pussy. Twisting and turning it, in and out, fast and deep, shoving it inside his wife; listening to the moans escaping her throat. As he continued fucking her with the dildo, she lifted her ass, encouraging him to continue. Lifting her ass then lowering herself, basically fucking the bed as he fucked her with the pseudo-dick.

"Please stop. I don't want this."

"You're sure acting like you want it. Fucking the bed, lifting your ass high in the air. This vibrator is so slippery I can barely hold it in place."

"Please stop. I don't want to come like this. I want you to be inside me."

"Now, that's something I'm open to. If I untie you, do you promise to be good?"

"Yes, yes. I promise. I just don't want to come this way. You know I love coming all over your dick. Please. Fuck me with your cock, and not this lame vibrator."

"How about a compromise? I won't fuck you with the vibrator anymore, but I'm also not going to untie your hands. I think I'll untie your feet instead. You've got to pay for the little attitude you gave me earlier. I think I'd like to fuck your ass. You think that's a fair compromise? Or punishment?"

"No. No, I don't think that's fair. I'd rather not. I'd rather you fuck my pussy."

"Yeah, well, I'd rather you not tease me in the shower, then turn me down. I think you need to feel my cock in your ass. Don't get me wrong. I do love how your pussy feels wrapped around my dick. Now, don't go anywhere while I slip a condom on." Ryan said teasing her. "I'll be taking your ass in just a minute."

"Please don't. I'm sorry. I had a rough day and I took it out on you. I'm sorry."

"Yeah, I know you're sorry. Thanks for the apology, wifey dear. But I'm still gonna fuck your ass."

With that, his wife began thrashing on the bed; doing her best to loosen the scarves holding her against her will. Ryan quickly slid the condom over his cock, anxious to feel her tightness engulf him. Grabbing the lube, he generously bathed his prick, and then slid a slippery finger into her puckered hole.

"I told you to stop!" She hissed. "Get your finger away from me, and keep your dick away from my ass." She screamed, kicking at him, trying her best to guard her rosette from his impending invasion. She clamped her legs together with the power of a vise grip, thanks to the exercise classes she took every other night.

"Baby, that's not going to stop me." He straddled her

legs, gently pulling her ass cheeks apart, eyeing the prize that would soon be his.

"I'm warning you! This is the last time I'm gonna say it. Get your fucking dick away from my ass!"

"Darling, I love it when you threaten me. Sweet, innocent teacher -- using such profanity. Naughty girl. Now, close that gorgeous mouth of yours and get ready to be fucked."

Ryan eased forward, targeting her rosette. As she had so many times before, Amy spread her legs, permitting him to enter her, as the urge to have her ass probed became overwhelming. It refused his entry at first, but he kept pressing forward until it finally gave in, accepting his dick as an unwanted visitor. "Damn, you're tight."

Ryan slowly plunged deep inside her, as she received his length with a sigh and a small moan; lifting her ass, signaling him to continue his intrusion. He entered her stretched opening, again and again, driving into her; slow and easy at first, then picking up the pace as she adjusted to his forceful thrusting. They fucked with a surge of passion. He watched his swollen member slowly disappear, and reappear, from her dark tunnel. Amy looked back, smiling her sinfully sexy grin.

"Enjoying yourself?"

Feeling like a kid with his hand caught in the cookie jar, Ryan replied, "I sure am, sweetness. I love the view from here."

Amy closed her eyes, spreading her legs, and pulling herself onto all fours, she shoved against her husband, matching his thrust with her own need. Ryan pushed against her round bottom, savoring the feeling of her ass accepting him. His hard cock slid easily in and out as he held her hips, listening to the smacking sound of their bodies as they collided.

"Yes. That's it. Fuck my ass. Punish me. Oh, so good. So fucking good." Amy muttered, unable to control the vixen that had been unleashed.

Ryan reached under her, wanting to increase her arousal further. He pressed his thumb against her clit and rubbed aggressively until he heard her moaning, knowing her orgasm was within reach. As they continue their tryst, he noticed her hands had become untied and she was gripping the sheets, pulling them to her as he took her from behind.

Finally, Ryan gently withdrew. Tossing the condom on the floor, he rolled her over to face him, pressing their bodies together and getting as much skin to skin contact as possible. Amy pulled her husband to her, holding his face in her hands as he pumped into her pussy. The angle was perfect, causing just enough friction to rub her clit. They gazed into each other's eyes as he slid in and out with almost painful slowness.

Amy raised her legs and locked them around Ryan's waist, encouraging him. He reached down, cupping her bottom and pressing farther inside her. She kissed him hard, sucking his tongue into her mouth, as he raised one hand to the back of her head, pulling her to him, and holding her by the hair. Ryan held her wanton body against his burning flesh, picking up the tempo as she embraced him, using their bodies as leverage to pound harder and fuck faster. Passion exploded inside them both as they rode the waves together. Amy writhed wildly underneath him as he directed his efforts at keeping himself ground into her aching pussy. She shook her head from side-to-side rocking her hips, matching him thrust for thrust.

"Lie back. Lie back so I can ride you."

Ryan did as he was told and lay down, allowing her to do whatever she needed. Amy moved to his head, straddling his face, and lowering herself onto his waiting tongue. He began licking her pussy, enjoying the juices that smeared his face. Ryan greedily sucked her clit, flicking it, knowing that was what she needed to get off. After only minutes, Amy began the familiar moans, growling louder as her orgasm raced through her body. At the height of her pleasure, she practically howled, dripping pussy juice around his lips and covering his face with her lubrication.

As she recovered, she lowered her body lying beside him momentarily before moving to take his dick in her hungry mouth. Amy sucked gently at first, and then with more fervor; deep-throating the shaft, causing Ryan's toes to curl as she glided her tongue around the cockhead; licking up and down the shaft and leaving a glistening trail from the moistness of her tongue. Just as she reached the top, she gobbled the length down to the base, then up again. Using her hands, she stroked him in unison with her mouth, squeezing the base as she rose up; wrapping her tongue around the tip in a nasty combination that brought him to the edge within minutes. Her gifted mouth worked his rod until he found himself pumping upward, encouraging her to suck him.

"Make me come. Yes, suck me. That's it. I want to come in your mouth. Don't stop."

She stroked her husband faster, squeezing his cock as she slurped his dick, until he felt the beginning of his orgasm. Ryan pumped into her mouth, then released spurt after spurt, draining himself; watching as she swallowed his seed, then wiped her mouth with her fingers, provocatively licking each one clean. Collapsing beside him, Amy turned. Smiling she mumbled, "Thank you. I so needed that! You always know what I need before I do. That, my dear husband, is why I love you and why I married you."

"You're welcome and thank you too. I needed it just as badly as you did. It's hard to believe that being a teacher and a police officer could be stressful. We really need to take a vacation."

"Sweetness, that would be fantastic. Do you think we really could? Just the two of us. What about the girls? We can't go on vacation without the girls. They deserve a treat too."

"How about we take the girls on a weekend trip to Disney? We could take them right after school lets out in six weeks. Then we could take a romantic vacation, just the two of us. Whatdaya think?"

"Oooh. I love that idea. A long weekend for the girls,

and then a week-long trip for us. Sounds terrific. Where do you think we should go? San Francisco? New York City? Phoenix? Maybe we could take a train through the Northwest? I'm so excited. We haven't been on a vacation since our honeymoon. We need to go someplace really fun. Maybe somewhere we can really let ourselves loose. Get a little wild," she teased, thrilled with the prospect of a week-long vacation.

"One of the officers in the department took his wife on a cruise. They went to a few places in the Caribbean. You think you'd like to go to the Caribbean?"

"The Caribbean? I've never been to the Caribbean. Do we need passports? We don't have passports. How long does it take to get a passport?" She rambled on, her mind racing with questions, the excitement of their proposed vacation practically making her hyper.

"First, yes, we need passports. And no -- we don't have them, but it only takes a trip to the post office and about a month for them to arrive. As for the Caribbean, I've never been. The guy from work mentioned they went to Mexico on their cruise. I think it'd be great to visit a foreign country. Even if that country is connected to the U.S." he joked, getting excited by the idea of a Mexican vacation. "Now, what are your thoughts about cruising? We could fly to Mexico if you prefer."

"You know I'm not crazy about flying. I think I'd like to try the cruise. A week on a boat with no worries.

No cooking, no cleaning, pools and hot tubs, room service, lounging in the sun reading a romance novel or two, maybe some erotica. Oooh. Sounds like so much fun. Maybe we get a little wild, try something a little naughty. You game?"

"Hell yeah, I'm game. I think a cruise is the perfect solution to our stress. Why don't you check the internet, gather some information, and we'll make some plans. Sound good?"

"Sounds perfect. Now, how about we start round two. I still want to ride your glorious cock, and I've got a few more orgasms left in me."

The End
~ Want More? ~

Ryan and Amy's story continues...
Seascape (Ryan and Amy's cruise where they fulfill a few sexual fantasies)

About the Author

I've been a military wife, a policeman's wife, a contractor's wife, and a security officer's wife; all while being married to the same man for almost twenty years. Over the years, I've learned a thing or two about keeping romance alive and the sex smoking hot. I love sex and I like helping others maximize their sexual pleasure which is why I've written and published a dozen erotic stories. I enjoy hearing from my fans so if you have suggestions, questions, or comments please contact me. Enjoy the heat! Laina   lainacharleston@yahoo.com

Made in the USA
Lexington, KY
19 December 2012